DO IT YOURSELF HOMEMADE FACE MASK

By Johnson Pfizer

Table of Contents

Introduction 4

Chapter 1 6
    What is Face mask? 6
    Uses of Face Mask 6
    When to Wear face mask? 7
    Types of Face Mask 8
    The right way to wear and remove face mask? 10

Chapter 2 13
    Masks management 13
    Comparing Surgical Masks and Surgical N95 Respirators 14
    N95 Respirators in Industrial and Health Care Settings 15
    Can face coverings prevent the spread of the virus? 16

Chapter 3 18
    What about homemade masks? 18
    How often do I need to wash it? 18
    Would a scarf work? 19
    Do masks confer any other benefits? 19

Chapter 4 21
    How to make your own Face mask 21
    What is FFP protection classes 21
    The importance of Filtering Facepieces respiratory protection 22
    How does a respirator mask work? 22
    FFP1 23
    FFP2 23
    FFP3 24
    How to do Your homemade face mask? 24
    Homemade face mask type 1 26

    Homemade face mask type 2 28
    Homemade face mask type 3 36
    Homemade face mask type 4 40
    Homemade face mask type 5 50
    Three ways to upgrade the mask 56
    Some things to remember about your homemade mask 57
Conclusion 57

Introduction

Wearing a face mask in public areas may impede the spread of an infectious disease by preventing both the inhalation of infectious droplets and their subsequent exhalation
and dissemination. In the event of a pandemic involving an airborne-transmissible agent, the general public will have limited access to the type of high- level respiratory protection worn by health care workers, such as N95 respirators. Images of members of the public wearing surgical masks were often used to illustrate the 2009 H1N1 flu pandemic. However, the evidence of proportionate benefit from widespread use of face masks is unclear.

A recent prospective cluster-randomized trial comparing surgical masks and non-fit-tested P2 masks (filters at least 94% of airborne particles) with no mask use in the prevention of influenza-like illness. The findings of the study found that adherence to mask use significantly reduced (95%) the risk for infection associated with influenza-like illness which include the just discovered Covid-19, but that less than 50% of participants wore masks most of the time.

Facemasks may prevent contamination of the work space during the outbreak of influenza or other droplet-spread communicable disease by reducing aerosol transmission. They may also be used to reduce the risk of body fluids, including blood, secretions, and excretions, from reaching the wearer's mouth and nose.

To date, studies on the efficacy and reliability of face masks have concentrated on their use by health care workers. Although health care workers are likely to be one of the highest risk groups in terms of exposure,they are also more likely to be trained in the use of masks and fit tested than the general public. Should the supply of standard commercial face masks not meet demand, it would be useful to know whether improvised masks could provide any protection to others from those who are infected and that include homemade face mask.

In this ebook we will discuss more on the uses of face mask and every other things you must know about the benefit of homemade face mask as well as how to make a good and affordable face mask for you and your family.

Wearing a medical mask is one of the prevention measures to limit spread of certain respiratory diseases, including 2019-nCoV, in affected areas. However, the use of a mask alone is insufficient to provide the adequate level of protection and other equally relevant measures should be adopted.If masks are to be used, this measure must be combined with hand hygiene and other IPC measures to prevent the human-to-human transmission of 2019-nCov.WHO has developed guidance for home care band health care settings con infection prevention and control(IPC) strategies for use when infection with 2019-nCoV is suspected. Wearing medical masks when not indicated may cause unnecessary cost, procurement burden and create a false sense of security that can lead to neglecting other essential measures such as hand hygiene practices.Furthermore, using a mask incorrectly may hamper its effectiveness to reduce the risk of transmission.

Chapter 1

What is Face mask?

A face mask is a device that you wear over your face, for example to prevent yourself from breathing bad air or from spreading germs, or to protect your face when you are in a dangerous situation.

Face masks are one tool utilized for preventing the spread of disease. They may also be called dental, isolation, laser, medical, procedure, or surgical masks. Face masks are loose-fitting masks that cover the nose and mouth, and have ear loops or ties or bands at the back of the head. There are many different brands and they come in different colors. It is important to use a face mask approved by the FDA.

Wearing a face mask is certainly not an iron-clad guarantee that you won't get sick – viruses can also transmit through the eyes and tiny viral particles, known as aerosols, can penetrate masks. However, masks are effective at capturing droplets, which is a main transmission route of coronavirus, and some studies have estimated a roughly fivefold protection versus no barrier alone (although others have found lower levels of effectiveness).

If you are likely to be in close contact with someone infected, a mask cuts the chance of the disease being passed on. If you're showing symptoms of coronavirus, or have been diagnosed, wearing a mask can also protect others. So masks are crucial for health and social care workers looking after patients and are also recommended for family members who need to care for someone who is ill – ideally both the patient and carer should have a mask.

However, masks will probably make little difference if you're just walking around town or taking a bus so there is no need to bulk-buy a huge supply.

Uses of Face Mask

Face mask provides a physical barrier to fluids and large particle droplets. Surgical mask is a type of face mask commonly used. When used properly, surgical masks can prevent infections transmitted by respiratory droplets.

Since the beginning of the global coronavirus pandemic, Americans have been told by the Centers for Disease Control and Prevention not to wear masks unless they are sick, caring for a sick person who is unable to wear one or working in health care.

Numerous reasons have been given: that they don't offer significant protection from germs, that the most effective models need special fitting in order to work, that regular people don't typically wear them correctly, that they'll give people a false sense of security and cause them to be lax about hand-washing and social distancing.
And most of all: that there aren't enough masks and respirators for the health-care workers who desperately need them so leave the masks to them.

Now there are big changes to that policy.

The Trump administration announced Friday that the CDC is now recommending people consider wearing cloth face coverings in public settings where other social distancing measures are difficult to maintain. Mayors in New York City and Los Angeles have already offered similar advice to citizens. In this ebook we are still going to discuss about cloth face mask and its efficiency.

There's one big reason for the change: There is increasing evidence that virus and other influenza can be spread by presymptomatic and asymptomatic carriers.

These new policies come with the vital plea that people don't use the medical-grade masks that are in short supply in hospitals. That means one thing: The era of the homemade masks and face coverings is upon us.

With this new attitude come many questions — which we'll attempt to answer here.

When to Wear face mask?

The purpose of all of us wearing face coverings or surgical masks anywhere people congregate is first and foremost to protect others if we sneeze or cough. These coverings will stop much of the large droplets that could otherwise reach people as far away as 18 feet away. Just-published research indicates that surgical masks can also decrease the amount of aerosolized virus the people produce by breathing and talking.

A big question is: Can these DIY or surgical masks also protect the wearer? The same research study shows these masks impede aerosolized virus being expelled out by the user so presumably they can decrease breathing in the virus, influenza or any other causative agent as well. But they aren't foolproof. These coverings don't fit the face tightly, so aerosolized virus and larger droplets can be sucked in through the gaps between the face and the mask when we take a breath.

Additionally, some of the viral particles are so small that they can be inhaled through the cloth or paper that's used to make these masks. People should not be lulled into a false sense of security in thinking that these types of masks will protect them from airborne, aerosolized virus especially in poorly ventilated spaces frequented by others. The best thing to do is to either avoid such spaces or be in them for as short a period of time as possible.

Wearing face coverings is recommended and requested for when you are indoors, including mass transit and ride-shares, with other people.

Anywhere you go, maintain physical distancing of at least 6 feet with no bodily contact. If someone nearby sneezes or coughs and they aren't wearing a mask, get at least 20 feet away, quickly. When you do go out on an errand, wear a face covering and get your business done as fast as you can.

You don't need an N95 mask if you wear a face covering when you go out in a public indoor place or ride mass transit and practice good physical distancing. Health care workers have to care for their patients within very close distances for prolonged periods of time. If they don't have an N95 mask, the risk goes way up for them.

Types of Face Mask

N95 respirators and surgical masks (face masks) are examples of personal protective equipment that are used to protect the wearer from airborne particles and from liquid contaminating the face. Centers for Disease Control and Prevention (CDC) National Institute for Occupational Safety and Health (NIOSH) and Occupational Safety and Health Administration (OSHA) also regulate N95 respirators.

It is important to recognize that the optimal way to prevent airborne transmission is to use a combination of interventions from across the hierarchy of controls,

Surgical Masks (Face Masks)

A surgical mask is a disposable medical device that can be bought in pharmacy and that protects against infectious agents transmitted by "droplets." These droplets can be droplets of saliva or secretions from the upper respiratory tract when the wearer exhales.

If worn by the caregiver, the surgical mask protects the patient and his or her environment (air, surfaces, equipment, surgical site). If worn by a contagious patient, it prevents the patient from contaminating his or her surroundings and environment. These masks should not be worn for more than 3 to 8 hours.

A surgical mask can also protect the wearer from the risk of splashes of biological fluids. In this case, the surgical mask must have a waterproof layer. It can also be equipped with a visor to protect the eyes.

But a surgical mask does not protect against "airborne" infectious agents so it will not prevent the wearer from being potentially contaminated by a virus such as the coronavirus.

A surgical mask is a loose-fitting, disposable device that creates a physical barrier between the mouth and nose of the wearer and potential contaminants in the immediate environment. Surgical masks are regulated under 21 CFR 878.4040. Surgical masks are not to be shared and may be labeled as surgical, isolation, dental, or medical procedure face masks. They may come with or without a face shield. These are often referred to as face masks, although not all face masks are regulated as surgical masks.

Surgical masks are made in different thicknesses and with different ability to protect you from contact with liquids. These properties may also affect how easily you can breathe through the face mask and how well the surgical mask protects you.

If worn properly, a surgical mask is meant to help block large-particle droplets, splashes, sprays, or splatter that may contain germs (viruses and bacteria), keeping it from reaching your mouth and nose. Surgical masks may also help reduce exposure of your saliva and respiratory secretions to others.

While a surgical mask may be effective in blocking splashes and large-particle droplets, a face mask, by design, does not filter or block very small particles in the air that may be transmitted by coughs, sneezes, or certain medical procedures. Surgical masks also do not provide complete protection from germs and other contaminants because of the loose fit between the surface of the face mask and your face.

Surgical masks are not intended to be used more than once. If your mask is damaged or soiled, or if breathing through the mask becomes difficult, you should remove the face mask, discard it safely, and replace it with a new one. To safely discard your mask, place it in a plastic bag and put it in the trash. Wash your hands after handling the used mask.

N95 Respirators
An N95 respirator is a respiratory protective device designed to achieve a very close facial fit and very efficient filtration of airborne particles.

The 'N95' designation means that when subjected to careful testing, the respirator blocks at least 95 percent of very small (0.3 micron) test particles. If properly fitted, the filtration capabilities of N95 respirators exceed those of face masks. However, even a properly fitted N95 respirator does not completely eliminate the risk of illness or death.

The right way to wear and remove face mask?

People should wear a surgical mask when they have respiratory infection; when taking care of patient with respiratory infection; or when visiting clinics or hospitals during pandemic or peak season for influenza in order to reduce the spread of infection.

Points to note on wearing a Face mask:
(a) Choose the appropriate mask size. Child size is available for selection as indicated.
(b) Perform hand hygiene before putting on a surgical mask.
(c) The surgical mask should fit snugly over the face:
(i) Most surgical masks adopt a three-layer design (Annex I) which includes an outer fluid-repelling layer, a middle layer serves as a barrier to germs, and an inner moisture-absorbing layer. Mask without the above functions is not recommended as it cannot provide adequate protection against infectious diseases transmitted by respiratory droplets. Wearer should follow the manufacturers' recommendations when using surgical mask, including proper storage and procedures of putting on surgical mask (e.g. determine which side of the mask is facing outwards). In general, the coloured side/the side with folds facing downwards of the surgical mask should face outwards with the metallic strip uppermost.

(ii) For tie-on surgical mask, secure upper ties at the crown of head. Then secure lower ties at the nape. For ear-loops type, position the elastic bands around both ears.

(iii) Extend the surgical mask to fully cover mouth, nose and chin(Image 3).

(iv) Mould the metallic strip over nose bridge and the surgical mask should fit snugly over the face(Image 4).

(d) Avoid touching the surgical mask after wearing. Otherwise, should perform hand hygiene before and after touching the mask.

(e) When taking off tie-on surgical mask, unfasten the ties at the nape first; then unfasten the ties at the crown of head(image 5). For ear-loops type, hold both the ear loops and take-off gently from face.

Avoid touching the outside of surgical mask during taking-off as it may be covered with germs.

(f) After taking off the surgical mask, discard in a lidded rubbish bin and perform hand hygiene immediately.

(g) Change surgical mask timely. In general, surgical mask should not be reused. Replace the mask immediately if it is damaged or soiled.

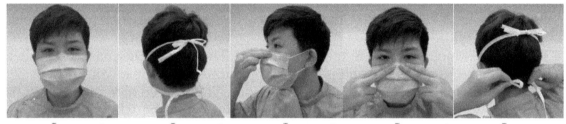

Image 1   Image 2   Image 3   Image 4   Image 5

Before putting on a mask, clean hands with alcohol-based hand rub or soap and water.

Cover mouth and nose with mask and make sure there are no gaps between your face and the mask.

Avoid touching the mask while using it; if you do, clean your hands with alcohol-based hand rub or soap and water.

Replace the mask with a new one as soon as it is damp and do not re-use single-use masks.

To remove the mask: remove it from behind (do not touch the front of mask); discard immediately in a closed bin; clean hands with alcohol-based hand rub or soap and water.

Additional Recommendations on Use of Surgical Mask during Influenza Pandemic in the Community Setting

During Influenza Pandemic, apart from using surgical mask properly, we should adopt the following preventive measures vigilantly to minimize the risk of getting infection:
(a)Perform hand hygiene frequently and properly.
(b)Perform hand hygiene before touching eyes, nose and mouth.
(c)Maintain respiratory etiquette/cough manners(Picture below).
(d)Stay at home if got sick and minimize contact with others.
(e)Stay away from possible sources of infection:(i)Minimize unnecessary social contacts and avoid visiting crowded places. If this is necessary, minimize the length of stay whenever possible. Moreover, person at a high risk of having infection-related complications, e.g. pregnant woman or persons with chronic illnesses are advised to wear surgical mask.
(ii)Avoid close contact with the infected persons.

How to put on other type of face mask

Clean your hands with soap and water or hand sanitizer before touching the mask.
Remove a mask from the box and make sure there are no obvious tears or holes in either side of the mask.
Determine which side of the mask is the top. The side of the mask that has a stiff bendable edge is the top and is meant to mold to the shape of your nose.
Determine which side of the mask is the front. The colored side of the mask is usually the front and should face away from you, while the white side touches your face.

Follow the instructions below for the type of mask you are using.
Face Mask with Ear loops: Hold the mask by the ear loops. Place a loop around each ear.
Face Mask with Ties: Bring the mask to your nose level and place the ties over the crown of your head and secure with a bow.
Face Mask with Bands: Hold the mask in your hand with the nosepiece or top of the mask at fingertips, allowing the headbands to hang freely below hands. Bring the mask to your nose level and pull the top strap over your head so that it rests over the crown of your head. Pull the bottom strap over your head so that it rests at the nape of your neck.

Mold or pinch the stiff edge to the shape of your nose.
If using a face mask with ties: Then take the bottom ties, one in each hand, and secure with a bow at the nape of your neck.
Pull the bottom of the mask over your mouth and chin.

How to remove other face mask

Clean your hands with soap and water or hand sanitizer before touching the mask. Avoid touching the front of the mask. The front of the mask is contaminated. Only touch the ear loops/ties/band. Follow the instructions below for the type of mask you are using.

Face Mask with Ear loops: Hold both of the ear loops and gently lift and remove the mask.

Face Mask with Ties: Untie the bottom bow first then untie the top bow and pull the mask away from you as the ties are loosened.

Face Mask with Bands: Lift the bottom strap over your head first then pull the top strap over your head.

Throw the mask in the trash. Clean your hands with soap and water or hand sanitizer.

Chapter 2

Masks management

If medical masks are worn, appropriate use and disposal is essential to ensure they are effective and to avoid any increase in risk of transmission associated with the incorrect use and disposal of masks. The following information on correct use of medical masks derives from the practices in health-care setting.

1. place mask carefully to cover mouth and nose and tie securely to minimise any gaps between the face and the mask;-while in use, avoid touching the mask; -remove the mask by using appropriate technique (i.e. do not touch the front but remove the lace from behind); -after removal or whenever you in advertently touch a used mask, clean hands by using an alcohol-based hand rubor soap and water if visibly soiled-replace masks with a new clean, dry mask as soon as they become damp/humid;-do not re-use single-use masks;-discard single-use masks after each use and dispose of them immediately upon removal. Cloth(e.g. cotton or gauze) masks are not recommended under any circumstance.

Comparing Surgical Masks and Surgical N95 Respirators

The FDA regulates surgical masks and surgical N95 respirators differently based on their intended use.

A surgical mask is a loose-fitting, disposable device that creates a physical barrier between the mouth and nose of the wearer and potential contaminants in the immediate environment. These are often referred to as face masks, although not all face masks are regulated as surgical masks. Note that the edges of the mask are not designed to form a seal around the nose and mouth.

An N95 respirator is a respiratory protective device designed to achieve a very close facial fit and very efficient filtration of airborne particles. Note that the edges of the respirator are designed to form a seal around the nose and mouth. Surgical N95 Respirators are commonly used in healthcare settings and are a subset of N95 Filtering Facepiece Respirators (FFRs), often referred to as N95s.

The similarities among surgical masks and surgical N95s are:
They are tested for fluid resistance, filtration efficiency (particulate filtration efficiency and bacterial filtration efficiency), flammability and biocompatibility. They should not be shared or reused.

General N95 Respirator Precautions
People with chronic respiratory, cardiac, or other medical conditions that make breathing difficult should check with their health care provider before using an N95 respirator because the N95 respirator can make it more difficult for the wearer to breathe. Some models have exhalation valves that can make breathing out easier and help reduce heat build-up. Note that N95 respirators with exhalation valves should not be used when sterile conditions are needed.

All FDA-cleared N95 respirators are labeled as "single-use," disposable devices. If your respirator is damaged or soiled, or if breathing becomes difficult, you should remove the respirator, discard it properly, and replace it with a new one. To safely discard your N95 respirator, place it in a plastic bag and put it in the trash. Wash your hands after handling the used respirator.

N95 respirators are not designed for children or people with facial hair. Because a proper fit cannot be achieved on children and people with facial hair, the N95 respirator may not provide full protection.

N95 Respirators in Industrial and Health Care Settings

Most N95 respirators are manufactured for use in construction and other industrial type jobs that expose workers to dust and small particles. They are regulated by the National Personal Protective Technology Laboratory (NPPTL) in the National Institute for Occupational Safety and Health (NIOSH), which is part of the Centers for Disease Control and Prevention (CDC)

However, some N95 respirators are intended for use in a health care setting. Specifically, single-use, disposable respiratory protective devices used and worn by health care personnel during procedures to protect both the patient and health care personnel from the transfer of microorganisms, body fluids, and particulate material. These surgical N95 respirators are class II devices regulated by the FDA, under 21 CFR 878.4040, and CDC NIOSH under 42 CFR Part 84.

N95s respirators regulated under product code MSH are class II medical devices exempt from 510(k) premarket notification, unless:

The respirator is intended to prevent specific diseases or infections, or
The respirator is labeled or otherwise represented as filtering surgical smoke or plumes, filtering specific amounts of viruses or bacteria, reducing the amount of and/or killing viruses, bacteria, or fungi, or affecting allergenicity, or
The respirator contains coating technologies unrelated to filtration (e.g., to reduce and or kill microorganisms).

Dental professionals should wear appropriate personal protective equipment—including masks, which adhere to Standard Precautions for protection of the mouth and nose—when splashes or sprays of blood and body fluids are likely.

Can face coverings prevent the spread of the virus?

The primary benefit of covering your nose and mouth is that you protect others. While there is still much to be learned about the novel coronavirus, it appears that many people who are infected are shedding the virus – through coughs, sneezes and other respiratory droplets – for 48 hours before they start feeling sick. And others who have the virus – up to 25%, according to Centers for Disease Control and Prevention Director Dr. Robert Redfield — may never feel symptoms but may still play a role in transmitting it.

That's why wearing a mask even if you don't feel sick can be a good idea.
If you cough or sneeze, the mask can catch those respiratory droplets so they don't land on other people or surfaces. "So it's not going to protect you, but it is going to protect your neighbor," says Dr. Daniel Griffin at Columbia University, an expert on infectious diseases. "If your neighbor is wearing a mask and the same thing happens, they're going to protect you. So masks worn properly have the potential to benefit people."

The best masks are N95 respirators, but the general public is urged not to use them because they are fiercely needed by health care workers right now. If you have those, consider donating them immediately to a local hospital or find a drop-off here. Same goes for surgical masks — those thin blue models-- which offer less protection but are helpful and are also in short supply.

If I'm wearing a mask and someone sneezes on me, would the mask offer some protection?
Yes. But only if you use the mask properly and don't touch it with your hands afterward.
Those droplets from a cough or sneeze would hit your mask instead of your mouth and nose — good news. But the next step is to take the mask off by the ear bands and either wash or discard it — without touching the front of it.

"That's what I see all the time," says Griffin. "That's why in the studies, masks fail — people don't use them [correctly]. They touch the front of it. They adjust it. They push it down somehow to get their nose stuck out."

If you touch the front of the mask, whatever that person coughed or sneezed on it is now on your hands.

As this video from the World Health Organization shows, you should take off your mask by removing the elastics or straps from behind your ears. Don't touch the front, and keep the mask away from your face.

One other thing: Ideally you would have eye protection, too, to keep that stranger's sneeze from getting in. Glasses and sunglasses aren't perfect but can help.

Chapter 3

What about homemade masks?

As NPR has previously reported, some research has shown that cotton T-shirt material and tea towels might help block respiratory droplets emitting from sick people — though it's not clear how much protection they provide.

Another study, of health care workers in Vietnam, found that use of cloth masks resulted in greater infection than either those wearing surgical masks or a control group, some of whom also wore surgical masks.

We don't yet know exactly how effective homemade masks are, but Griffin thinks they're a good idea — he has even taken to wearing one over his N95 respirator.

How often do I need to wash it?

Griffin says to think of a mask as like underwear: It needs to be washed after each use.
"You don't take this dirty mask off, put it in your purse and then stick it back on your face," he says. "It's something that once you put on, is potentially either touching your coughs, sneezes or the spray of your speech, or protecting you from the coughs, spray, speech of other people. And now it's dirty. It needs to basically be either discarded or washed."

So if you're wearing a cloth mask, put it into the laundry basket immediately. If it's disposable, throw it away.
It's a big no-no to pull the mask down to eat a snack, then pull it back up: You've just gotten whatever dirty stuff is on the mask on your hands and into your mouth.

Is there one best mask design?
There is little data so far on cloth or homemade masks in general — let alone data that dictates how many pleats to put on your home-sewn version.

Griffin says the best material to use is a tight-weave cotton. "Don't use a synthetic or a polyester because they've looked at the virus's ability to survive on surfaces, and spandex is the worst," he says.

Johns Hopkins Medicine has one design you might try. Kaiser Permanente has another design, as well as a video showing how to make a mask using a sewing machine. Both recommend 100% woven cotton fabric. Kaiser recommends washing and drying the fabric two or three times before cutting it, so it doesn't shrink later.

You can make a mask out of a T-shirt, no sewing machine required. You could also try making one out of (unused) shop towels. But no matter what you make it out of, try to make it fit closely to your face and don't touch the front of it once you've started wearing it.
If you use cloth masks, make a number of them so you can wear a fresh one each time you go out.

Would a scarf work?

Probably not as well as a mask that fits closely to your face.
"You can imagine if you put a loosely knit scarf with lots of holes in it ... that would not be very effective," says Dr. Michael Klompas, an infectious disease physician at Brigham and Women's Hospital.

The goal is to create a barrier that catches droplets and keeps others from coming in, so you want coverage that is tightly woven and close-fitting.

Do masks confer any other benefits?

Masks can also function as an important visual cue, says Joseph Allen, an assistant professor of exposure and assessment science at Harvard University T.H. Chan School of Public Health.

They're a "reminder that we need to be taking these precautions and serve as a reminder to people to keep that 6-foot buffer," he says. "It should be seen as a badge of honor. If I'm wearing a mask out in public, it means I'm concerned about you, I'm concerned about my neighbors, I'm concerned about strangers on the chance that I'm infectious. I want to do my part in limiting how I might impact you."

Klompas agrees — and says that it can also give the wearer a welcome sense of security.

"It feels like you're behind a shield," he says, "and I think that in itself can be reassuring."
And for the others around you, it's a warning. "It says: Watch out. There's a public health crisis right now, there's a virus going around, we need to be on top guard," says Klompas. "I think it can actually be a reinforcer, a reminder of the state of crisis that we face in society."

But he says that masks are not a replacement for all the other steps we need to take right now to protect ourselves from the coronavirus — especially social distancing and good hand hygiene.

Chapter 4

How to make your own Face mask

It's difficult to keep your distance in a grocery store or pharmacy during a pandemic such as the Covid-19, so now the CDC says we should wear a homemade mask in public to slow the spread of the coronavirus — particularly in areas with high community transmission.

Officials don't want healthy people using medical masks because of fears they would buy them all (kind of like toilet paper) and not leave them for health care workers.

We have the answer: Make your own.

The masks don't need to be professional-grade to help fight against airborne transmitted diseases such as Influenza and COVID-19. According to recent studies, the virus can spread between people in proximity by coughing, sneezing or even speaking.

It is important to note that covering your face with a piece of cloth won't protect you. But, it could help you from spreading the virus if you're like some people who lack symptoms and don't know they have it.

Sewing your own mask is easy, says Jeannette Childers, She's among scores of volunteers across the country sewing masks. So far, she's made so many for the Americans.

What is FFP protection classes

Aerosols and fine particles are two of the most treacherous health risks in a working environment and are nearly invisible in our breathing air. Filtering facepieces offer protection in three classes against these dangers: FFP1, FFP2 and FFP3.

Many dust masks bear the code FFP. This stands for 'filtering facepiece'. It shows what and how many particles of suspended dust, mist or fibres are filtered.

It isn't always easy to figure out all the different pictograms, standards and quality marks. With the right help, you can find the necessary information on every package so you always make the best choice at the building supply store. Always follow the instructions in the manual for correct use.

The importance of Filtering Facepieces respiratory protection

Dangerous particles can cause cancer or may be radioactive; others harm the respiratory system. Contact throughout decades may cause development of serious conditions. In the best case, all workers are confronted with are upsetting smells. Filtering facepieces offer protection in three classes against aqueous oily aerosols, smoke, and fine particles during work. Their protective function conforms to EU norm EN 149. This kind of facepiece is also known as particle-filtering half mask or fine particle mask and they are divided into the protection classes FFP1, FFP2 and FFP3.

How does a respirator mask work?

Filtering facepieces protect from respirable dust, smoke, and aqueous fog (aerosols), however they offer no protection from vapor and gas. The classifying system consists of the three FFP classes, the abbreviation FFP stands for "filtering facepiece". A respirator mask covers mouth and nose and is constructed of various filter materials and the mask itself. Their use is mandatory in working environments exceeding the occupational exposure limit value (OEL). This is the maximal concentration of dust, smoke, and/or aerosols in our breathing air that won't result in harm to health. In case of transgression, respirator masks must be worn.

Against what do respirator masks protect?

Depending on the total leakage and filtering of particle sizes up to 0.6 μm, respirator masks ranging from FFP1 through FFP2 to FFP3 offer breathing protection for various concentrations of pollutants. The total leakage comes about based on the filter penetration and leakages in the mouth and nose area. Our uvex respirator masks aim to avoid these by adapting our masks to human anatomy. Thanks to innovative filter technology, the breathing resistance can be held minimal and breathing isn't exacerbated intercepted particles in the filter after multiple-time wearing.

FFP1

- protection from atoxic and non-fibrogenic kinds of dust
- inhaling may result in development of health conditions; can also irritate the respiratory system and cause unpleasant odors
- total leakage may amount to a maximum of 25 %
- this kind of mask may be applied under a fourfold OEL transgression at the most

Protection class FFP1 respirator masks are made for working environments in which neither poisonous nor fibrogenic kinds of dust and aerosols are to be expected. They filter at least 80 % of the particles measuring up to 0.6 μm and may be worn as long as the maximum workplace concentration transgression measures no more than the fourfold value. The building or food industry put FFP1 respirator masks to use in many cases.

FFP2

- protection from firm and fluid deleterious kinds of dust, smoke, and aerosols
- particles may be fibrogenic – which means they irritate the respiratory system in the short term and can result in reduction of elasticity of pulmonary tissue in the long run
- total leakage may amount to a maximum of 11%
- OEL transgression to the tenfold value

Protection class FFP2 respirator masks are made for working environments in which deleterious and mutagenic particles can be found in the breathing air. Respirator masks of this class must contain at least 94 % of the particles measuring up to 0.6 μm and may be used in environments transgressing the OEL up to a maximum of the tenfold concentration. The same goes for the TRK value (technical reference concentration). Protection class FFP2 respirator masks are often worn in the metal and mining industry. Workers in these industries are frequently in contact with aerosols, fog and smoke that result in conditions of the respiratory system such as lung cancer in the long term. On top, they harbor the massive risk of secondary diseases and active tuberculosis of the lung. Our uvex filter system with a layer of carbon protects wearers from unpleasant odors on top of the required breathing protection.

FFP3

- protection from poisonous and deleterious kinds of dust, smoke, and aerosols
- when working with oncogenic or radioactive substances or pathogens such as viruses, bacteria and fungal spores FFP3-class respirator masks are recommended
- total leakage may amount to a maximum of 5%
- OEL transgression to the thirtyfold value

Protection class FFP3 respirator masks offer maximum protection from breathing air pollution. The total leakage may amount to a maximum of 5% and they must filter 99% of all particles measuring up to 0.6 μm. This kind of mask also filters poisonous, oncogenic and radioactive particles. Protection class FFP3 masks are used in working environments transgressing the OEL by the thirtyfold industry-specific values. They are often used in the chemistry industry.

How to do Your homemade face mask?

The masks don't need to be professional-grade to help fight against FLU and COVID-19. According to recent studies, the virus can spread between people in proximity by coughing, sneezing or even speaking.

It is important to note that covering your face with a piece of cloth won't protect you. But, it could help you from spreading the virus if you're like some people who lack symptoms and don't know they have it.

Sewing your own mask is easy, says Jeannette Childers, who's 77 and lives in Mesa, Arizona. She's among scores of volunteers across the country sewing masks. So far, she's made 65.

What type of ties do you want?

There are three main ways we recommend tying the mask to your face, and you'll want to plan it out before starting.

Ties that go around your ears. These are loose ties that you tie together behind your ears each time you put the mask on. This is simplest to make and requires the least work up front, but you'll need to tie the mask each time you wear it. You can't simply slip it on.

Ear loops. Elastic may be better than fabric for this style, since you'll need the ties to be short and tight enough to stay securely wrapped around your ears, but not so short and tight that they pop off.

Ties that go around the back of your head. You'll want the ties to be long enough to go around the back of your head horizontally, but short enough that the fit won't be too loose.

What you'll need
- Fabric. You'll need enough to make two 12″-by-6″ rectangles (the size of the template below.) Use a tightly woven fabric. Cotton-blend t-shirts and pillowcases are good bets.
- Scissors to cut the fabric.
- Something to tie the mask on. This could be elastic, strips of fabric, or something such as shoelaces.
- Needle and thread. If you don't have any, there are still options.

Homemade face mask type 1

Materials
Front: 100% unused cotton fabric—no metallic fabrics Back:100% unused cotton or cotton flannel Attachment:1/8", 1/4",or 3/8" flat elastic (white is preferred, black is OK) OR Four 15" x 1/4" inch bias-tape style ties (no raw edges, white/light preferred, black/dark OK

(Note:The instructions list three sizes: Small, Medium, and Large. We would recommend making Small-and Medium-sized masks primarily.
If possible, making a few Large masks would be helpful as well. See instructions for cutting sizes below.)

1)Cut two rectangles of fabric, one for the inside, one for the outside.
a. Small: 7.5 x 5inches
b. Medium: 9 x 6 inches
c. c.Large: 10 x 7 inches

2) Cut elastic or ties. All ties can be ¼" x 15". You will need 4 for each mask (one for each corner). Elastic should be cut as follows. You will need 2 pieces for each mask.
a. Small: 6.5 inches
b. Medium: 7 inches
C. Large: 7.5 inches
3) Put right sides of cotton mask fabric together.
4) Starting at the center of bottom (long) edge, sew to the first corner, stop. Sew a piece of elastic or a fabric tie into the corner. A few stitches forward and back will hold this.
5) Sew to the next corner, stop, and bring the other end of that same elastic to the corner and sew a few stitches forward and back.If you are using fabric ties, add a new tie.
6) Now sew across that top of the mask to the next corner. Again put a 7" length of elastic in the corner (or a new tie)
7) Sew to the next corner and sew in the other end of the same elastic (or a new tie).
8) Sew across the bottom leaving about 1.5" to 2" open. Stop, cut the thread.
9) Turn mask right-sideout.
10) Pin 3 tucks on each side of the mask. Make sure the tucks are in the same direction. There must be 3 tucks to ensure a tight fit on the face.
11) Sew around the edge of the mask twice.

12) When you have finished your masks, please use a Sharpie marker to mark a 1" tall S, M, or L on the lower left corner of the insideof each mask to indicate the size. This will help providers select the correct size. If you do not have a Sharpie, please somehow designate size for the masks before you drop them off.

Homemade face mask type 2

Supplies and tools
This is a relatively simple project so it doesn't require a lot of materials and tools to be completed. You need:

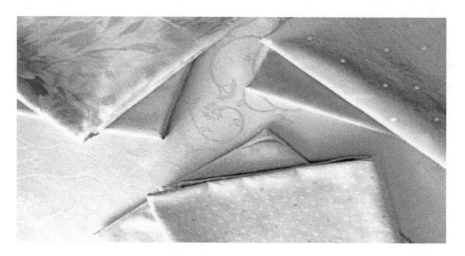

Face mask materials
- main fabric – about 13"x 7", cotton – all white or medical themed (tightly woven cotton, such as quilting cotton or cotton used in quality bed sheets)
- lining fabric about 13" x 6", cotton (tightly woven)
- filter (optional)
- 1/16" round elastic (preferable, currently available option , 1/8" or 1/4" flat elastic
- scissors (or better yet rotary cutter and a cutting mat)
- iron and ironing board
- sewing clips or pins
- a sewing machine (I recommend this one this one for beginners as it gets the work done and is reasonably priced or needle and a thread if you are handsewing

INSTRUCTIONS:
1. View the pattern and cut the fabric

face mask pattern and supplies on the cutting mat, Its original dimensions are 8.5 x 11 inches, which is about the size of a letter, small enough for easy printing. If you are not sure whether the dimensions are right, there is a small test square – 1 inch x 1 inch (US) and 2cm x2cm (for those outside US) on it so go ahead and measure it.

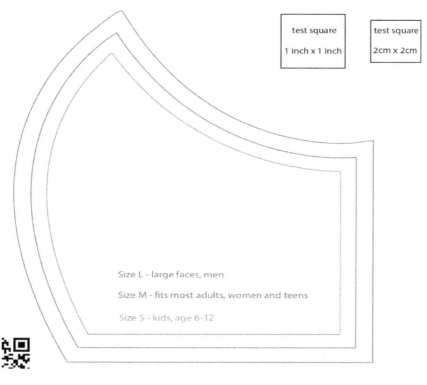

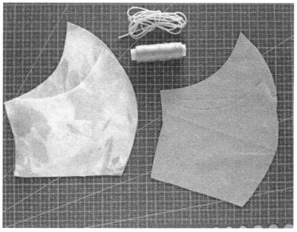

Download the pattern, print it out, and cut it accordingly. Before you put it onto your main fabric to cut it, fold the fabric in half so that the wrong sides are facing each other. Pin the pattern onto this folded fabric and cut the fabric just like the picture above.

DO IT YOURSELF HOMEMADE FACE MASK

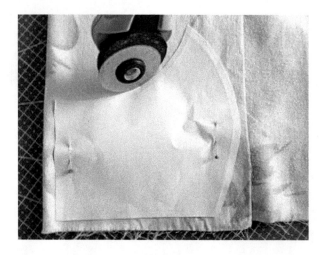

The seam allowance is 1/2 inch and is already included on all sides except for the ear side where you should add additional one inch seam allowance.

Repeat this step with the lining fabric as well. This time, however, do not add a seam allowance for the ear section.

TIPS: Several seamstresses asked us for fabric recommendations. Basically any thickly-woven cotton is fine and it is even better if you can add a filter medium

I saw someone wearing a stethoscope fabric mask and though that this is a great way to show appreciation to our front-liners. So, I found some suitable fabrics that can be purchased online. If you spot a great design, you can let your friends know

2. Sew the curve line of the face mask
Turn both pieces over and set them so that the right sides are on each other.
Sew along the curved line on both pieces.

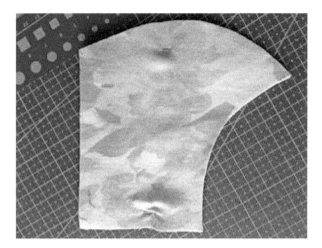

Then draw a line quarter-inch away from the original side line, on the inner layer. Do this for both side seams of the inner layer.

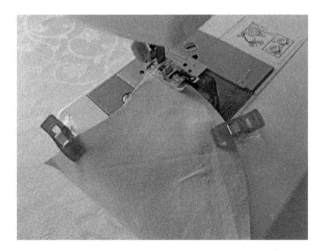

Next, you will need to clip the seam allowance on the curve part of the mask half an inch apart, both on the outer and the inner layer. Doing this allows the edge to stretch nicely instead of bulking up when you flip it inside out.

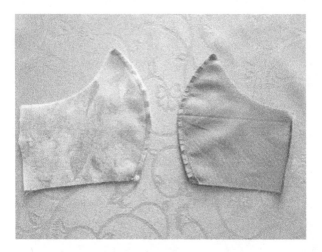

Now turn both pieces inside out and use the iron to press the seam allowances to different sides. If you want your mask to have a more professional look, topstitch near the seam line so that the seam allowances stay flat. Fold the side at the line you drew earlier and put the raw edge inside to hide it before topstitching it in place. Do this on each of the ear sides of the inner layer.

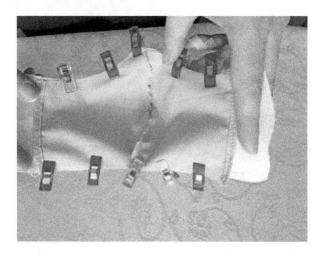

It's time to join the two layers together now. Put the inner layer on top of the outer, right sides facing each other so that the upper and lower edges align. Make a stitch at the bottom and top seam lines. If you did everything right up to this point, you will find that the edge of the outer layer is a about an inch away from the side seam line on the inner layer. If this isn't the case, retrace your steps and see where you made a mistake so that you can fix it.

Clip that curve on the seam allowance where the two layers meet and leave about half of an inch from the ends untouched. Flip the mask inside out again. Press the seams flat.

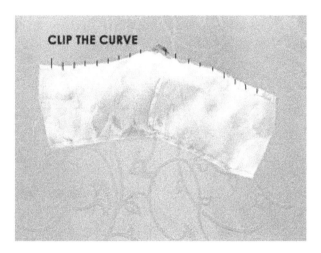

Fold the top and bottom raw edges of the outer layer twice and topstitch along the edge. Do this on the bottom seam line as well.

3. Add the elastic band and finalize your mask

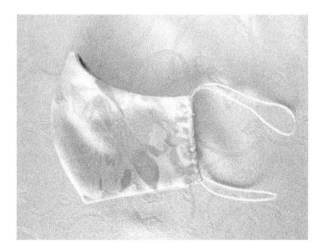

final face mask with elastic - ready to insert the filter
Now you will be making a channel for the elastic band. Fold the raw edge of the outer layer about a quarter of an inch away from the edge. Fold once again until that edge meets the edge of the inner layer.

Topstitch a vertical line across the part you just folded and you will be left with a vertical tube through which you can pull the elastic band.
– For 2 separate ear loops – you'll need 2 x 6"-8" of elastic for the adult sizes or 2 x 5 – 5 1/2" (kids)
– For one continuous piece that goes around the head – use 1 x 15-17" of elastic (again, depending on the size of the face)

TIP: Many makers report shortage of thin round elastic. You can use hair ties, ribbons or even make ties out of fabric.

4. Insert flexible nose wire (Optional)

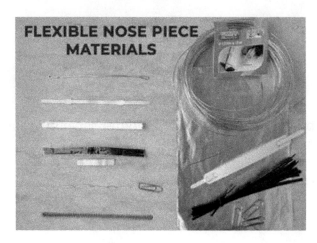

The mask will fit your face more closely if you add a flexible nose piece and mold it over your nose. I suggest using a 7" long crafting wire or couple of twist ties, but as those are not always available, we get creative.

We've compiled our ideas and feedback from our readers and got to work. We tested which are the most suitable materials and what is the best length for the nose piece. Here's what we found – the most suitable materials for nose wire.

5. Insert filter (optional) and use the mask

You will also notice an opening between the outer and inner layers. This is where you can put the filter in. Change it regularly and keep your mask clean by washing it in the washing machine after each use.
What to use as a FILTER.

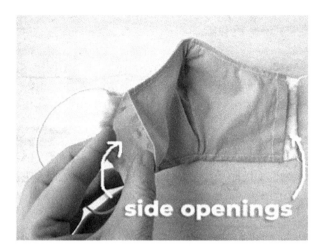

Note that these are not medically rated and their ability to protect is unknown:

As far as the filter goes you may use a piece of vacuum cleaner bag or HEPA filter without fiberglass, non woven fabric, or even an air-dried anti-bacterial wet wipe as filter. While those won't be able to stop the virus, they will be able to filter out more particles than fabrics alone. It probably all boils down to finding a balance between breath-ability and filtering. You'll have to make your own call here, and it would be smart to research whether and what filter to use.

Many readers asked why use vacuum dustbags as filter? According to this 2013 Cambridge university study which evaluated the capacity of several household materials to block bacterial and viral aerosols, vacuum cleaner bags were considered the most formidable household material with a rate of nearly 86 percent protection against the smallest particles they tested.

When placing the filter inside, make sure that it isn't crumbled up and that it reaches all the way to the upper edge. Once you put the mask on, make sure that it covers your nose well and that there are no gaps between your face and the mask.

Homemade face mask type 3

CDC recommends wearing cloth face coverings in public settings where other social distancing measures are difficult to maintain (e.g., grocery stores and pharmacies), especially in areas of significant community-based transmission.

CDC also advises the use of simple cloth face coverings to slow the spread of the virus and help people who may have the virus and do not know it from transmitting it to others. Cloth face coverings fashioned from household items or made at home from common materials at low cost can be used as an additional, voluntary public health measure.

Cloth face coverings should not be placed on young children under age 2, anyone who has trouble breathing, or is unconscious, incapacitated or otherwise unable to remove the mask without assistance.

The cloth face coverings recommended are not surgical masks or N-95 respirators. Those are critical supplies that must continue to be reserved for healthcare workers and other medical first responders, as recommended by current CDC guidance.

Sewn Cloth Face Covering
Supplies needed to create a cloth face covering are displayed. The supplies pictured include: one sewing machine, one twelve-inch ruler, one pencil, two six inch pieces of elastic string, two rectangle pieces of cotton cloth, 1 sewing needle, 1 bobby pin, 1 spool of thread, and 1 pair of scissors.

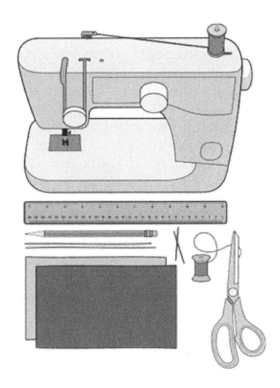

Materials

- Two 10"x6" rectangles of cotton fabric
- Two 6" pieces of elastic (or rubber bands, string, cloth strips, or hair ties)
- Needle and thread (or bobby pin)
- Scissors
- Sewing machine

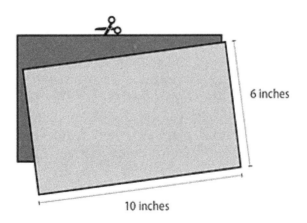

DO IT YOURSELF HOMEMADE FACE MASK

Tutorial

1. Cut out two 10-by-6-inch rectangles of cotton fabric. Use tightly woven cotton, such as quilting fabric or cotton sheets. T-shirt fabric will work in a pinch. Stack the two rectangles; you will sew the mask as if it was a single piece of fabric.

A close up of the two rectangular pieces of cloth needed to make a cloth face covering is shown. These pieces of cloth have been cut using a pair of scissors. Each piece of cloth measures ten inches in width and six inches in length.

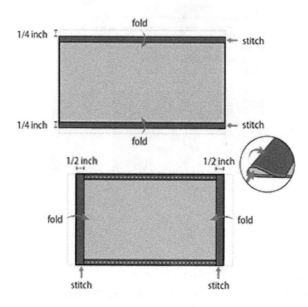

2. Fold over the long sides ¼ inch and hem. Then fold the double layer of fabric over ½ inch along the short sides and stitch down.

The top diagram shows the two rectangle cloth pieces stacked on top of each other, aligning on all sides. The rectangle, lying flat, is positioned so that the two ten inch sides are the top and the bottom of the rectangle, while the two six inch sides are the left and right side of the rectangle. The top diagram shows the two long edges of the cloth rectangle are folded over and stitched into place to create a one-fourth inch hem along the entire width of the top and bottom of the rectangle. The bottom diagram shows the two short edges of the cloth rectangle are folded over and stitched into place to create a one-half inch hem along the entire length of the right and left sides of the face covering.

DO IT YOURSELF HOMEMADE FACE MASK

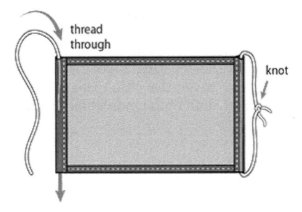

3. Run a 6-inch length of 1/8-inch wide elastic through the wider hem on each side of the mask. These will be the ear loops. Use a large needle or a bobby pin to thread it through. Tie the ends tight.
Don't have elastic? Use hair ties or elastic head bands. If you only have string, you can make the ties longer and tie the mask behind your head.

Two six inch pieces of elastic or string are threaded through the open one-half inch hems created on the left and right side of the rectangle. Then, the two ends of the elastic or string are tied together into a knot.

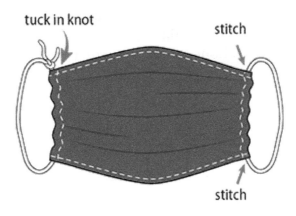

4. Gently pull on the elastic so that the knots are tucked inside the hem. Gather the sides of the mask on the elastic and adjust so the mask fits your face. Then securely stitch the elastic in place to keep it from slipping.

How to Wear an emergency Cloth Face Covering

Side view of an individual wearing a cloth face covering, which conceals their mouth and nose areas and has a string looped behind the visible ear to hold the covering in place. The top of the covering is positioned just below the eyes and the bottom extends down to cover the chin. The visible side of the covering extends to cover approximately half of the individual's cheek.

Cloth face coverings should :-

- fit snugly but comfortably against the side of the face
- be secured with ties or ear loops
- include multiple layers of fabric
- allow for breathing without restriction
- be able to be laundered and machine dried without damage or change to shape

Homemade face mask type 4

Assembly Guide Preparation
Fabric
This mask has two layers—the inner layer touching the face and the outer layer. The two layers can be made of the same fabric or different fabrics. Use 100% cotton or a cotton blend for the best filtration and breathability.
It takes two pieces of fabric about 14.5 in. x 7.5 in. (36 cm. x 18 cm.) to make one adult mask .

There are three sizes: Large, Medium, and Small. Patterns are available at the end of these instructions.

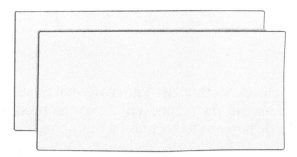

Ear Loop Material

Each mask needs two strips for ear loops. Ear loop material should be less than ½ inch (1.25 cm) wide. Some options are elastic, elastic cord, string, ribbon, bias tape, or even shoelaces.

If using elastic, each piece should be 12 inches (35.5 cm.) long. For other materials each piece should be 15 inches (38 cm) long.

Sewing Equipment

- Sewing machine
- Scissors or rotary cutter
- Thread
- Straight pins
- Safety pins

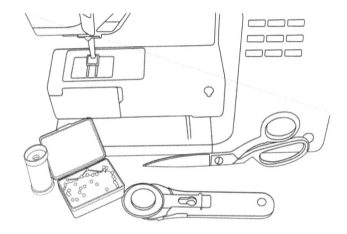

Work Area

Before you start sewing, ensure you are symptom free. Wash and sanitize your hands and your work area thoroughly with a disinfectant (it must indicate that it kills viruses) per the instructions on the label. Ensure there are no potential contaminants (e.g., pet hair, food, etc.) in the work area.

Assembly Guide Sewing Instructions

Step 1–Cut out the two main mask pieces.
- Fold the fabric in half. On the folded edge of the fabric, place the pattern edge marked "place on fold".
- Pin the pattern on the fold of the fabric and cut it out.

- Repeat step 1 to cut the second piece.

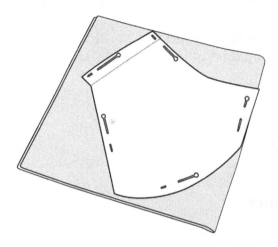

Step 2 – Make the chin part of the mask.
- Open one of the cutout mask pieces. Fold it in half on the fold line, with the right sides inside.
- Sew along the chin seam, stitching 1/4 in (0.7 cm) from the edge.
- If desired, press the seam to the side to help it lay flat.
- Fold and sew the second mask piece in the same way.

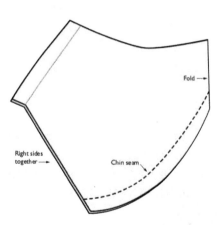

Step 3 – Join the inner and outer layers together.
- Lay the two mask pieces on top of each other, with right sides of the fabric together.

- Sew the two layers together across the top of the mask, using a ¼ in (0.7 cm) seam.
- Sew the two layers together across the bottom of the mask.

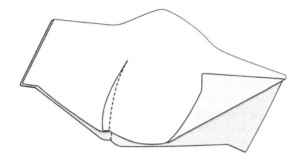

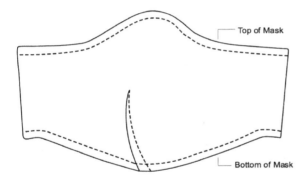

Step 4–Turn the mask right-side out.
- Press with an iron.

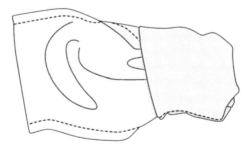

Step 5–Topstitch along the top and bottom edges.
- Keep your stitching close to the edges.

- Do not stich across the sides of the mask.

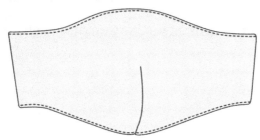

Step 6–Make the casing (a hollow channel) for the ear loop to go through.

On each side:
- Fold the raw side edges toward the inside of the mask about ¼ in (0.7 cm) (See Figure 10).
- Then fold over again, about 5/8 in (1.5 cm).
- Pin in place and stitch.

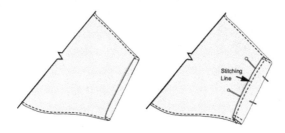

Step 7–Thread the ear loop through the casing along the sides of the mask.

- Use a large-eye plastic needle or attach the end of the elastic to a small safety pin. Push the elastic through the casing on both sides of the mask.

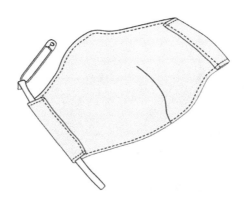

Step 8–Make loops the right size.
•Tie the loop ends loosely. The wearer can adjust the length by tying a knot.

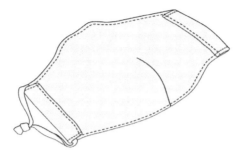

Large Face Mask

Sew with 1/4 in (6 mm) seam allowance.

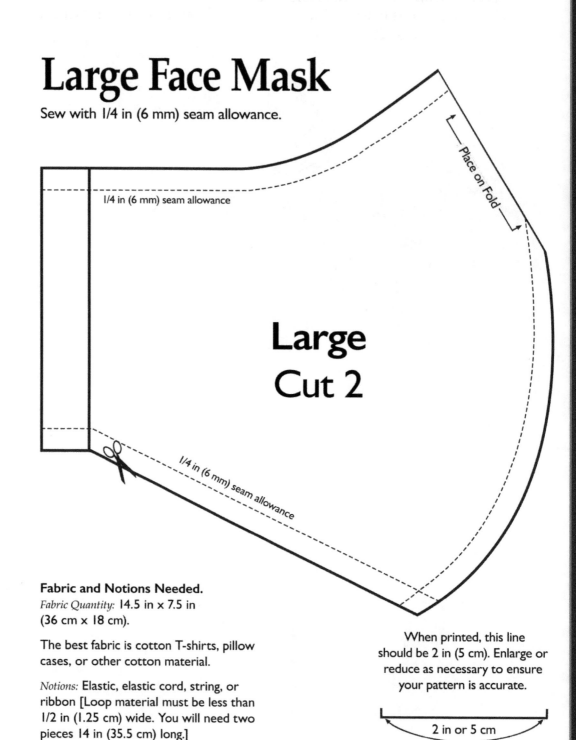

Fabric and Notions Needed.
Fabric Quantity: 14.5 in x 7.5 in (36 cm x 18 cm).

The best fabric is cotton T-shirts, pillow cases, or other cotton material.

Notions: Elastic, elastic cord, string, or ribbon [Loop material must be less than 1/2 in (1.25 cm) wide. You will need two pieces 14 in (35.5 cm) long.]

When printed, this line should be 2 in (5 cm). Enlarge or reduce as necessary to ensure your pattern is accurate.

2 in or 5 cm

Medium Face Mask

Sew with 1/4 in (6 mm) seam allowance

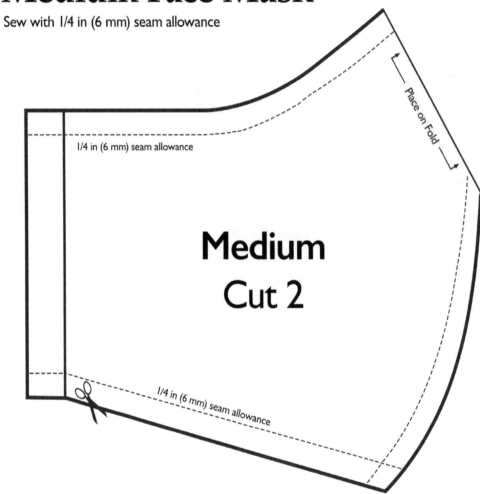

Fabric and Notions Needed.

Fabric Quantity: 14.5 in x 7.5 in (36 cm x 18 cm).

The best fabric is cotton T-shirts, pillow cases, or other cotton material.

Notions: Elastic, elastic cord, string, or ribbon [Loop material must be less than 1/2 in (1.25 cm) wide. You will need two pieces 14 in (35.5 cm) long.]

When printed, this line should be 2 in (5 cm). Enlarge or reduce as necessary to ensure your pattern is accurate.

2 in or 5 cm

Small Face Mask

Sew with 1/4 in (6 mm) seam allowance

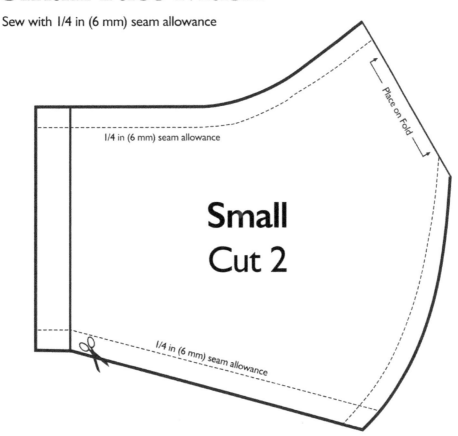

1/4 in (6 mm) seam allowance

Place on Fold

Small Cut 2

1/4 in (6 mm) seam allowance

Fabric and Notions Needed.

Fabric Quantity: 14.5 in x 7.5 in (36 cm x 18 cm).

The best fabric is cotton T-shirts, pillow cases, or other cotton material.

Notions: Elastic, elastic cord, string, or ribbon [Loop material must be less than 1/2 in (1.25 cm) wide. You will need two pieces 14 in (35.5 cm) long.]

When printed, this line should be 2 in (5 cm). Enlarge or reduce as necessary to ensure your pattern is accurate.

2 in or 5 cm

DO IT YOURSELF HOMEMADE FACE MASK

Homemade face mask type 5

MATERIALS:
You will need:
- 1.2 pieces of 100% cotton fabric 7" x 9"
- 2.2 pieces of 100% cotton fabric 1 ½" x 6"
- 3.2 pieces of 100% cotton fabric 1 ½" x 40"
- 4.Ruler
- 5.Pins
- 6.Scissors
- 7.Sewing machine & thread

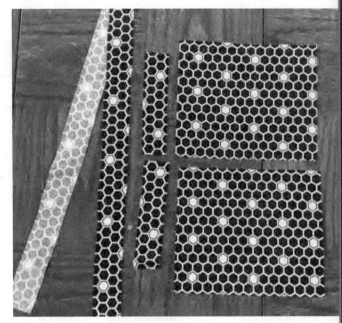

Masks should be constructed from tightly woven, high thread count cotton fabrics. The fabric should not have any stretch, and should not be knit (i.e. t-shirt material).
Recommended fabrics include: Poplin, Shirting, Sateen, and Percale in 100% cotton. A possible source of fabric is high thread count sheets and pillow cases.

Wondering if your fabric will work? A simple way to check is to fold it into two layers. You shouldn't be able to see through the fabric, but you should still be able to breathe if you hold it over your mouth.

Before you start, fabrics should be washed and dried on Hot in order to pre-shrink them.

INSTRUCTIONS:
1.Lay main mask pieces wrong sides together. Sew around edges at 1/4" to secure

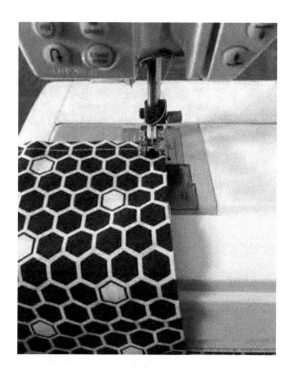 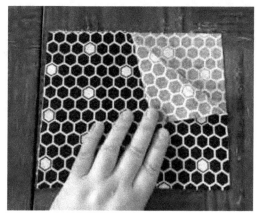

2. To create pleats: place pins along 7" edges as illustrated
3. Bring first needle to second to create pleat. Repeat with third & forth, fifth & sixth
4. Sew along previous stitching to secure pleats

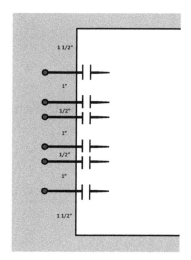

DO IT YOURSELF HOMEMADE FACE MASK

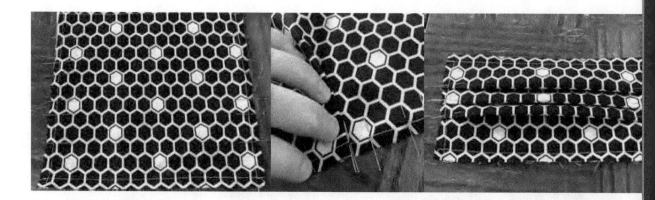

5. Press up 1/4" on both 1 ½" x 6" binding pieces

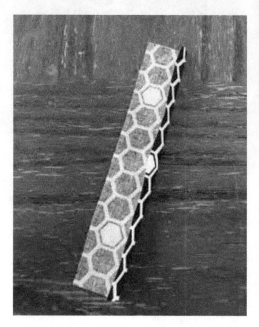

6. Lay unfolded side along pleated edge of mask, stitch at

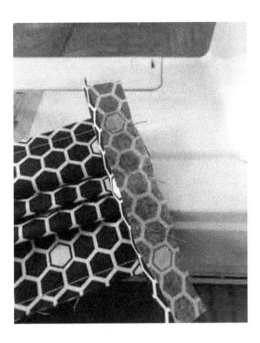

7. Fold binding around seam allowance & pin on opposite side, encasing raw edge. Topstitch in place.

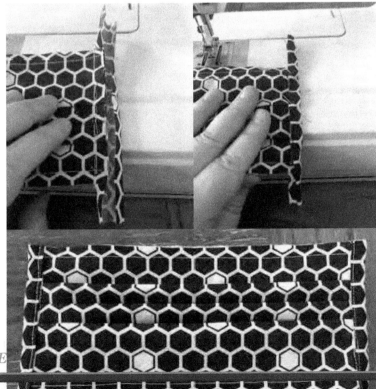

8. Repeat for opposite side. Trim binding to match mask

9. On both 1 ½" x 40" strap pieces, fold & press long edges to center
10. Fold the mask in half along the long edge & mark the center with a pin. Do the same with the strap
11. Matching centers, pin the strap in place. Stitch to mask body at 1/4" 12. Wrap strap around seam allowance as on binding & pin

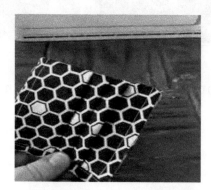

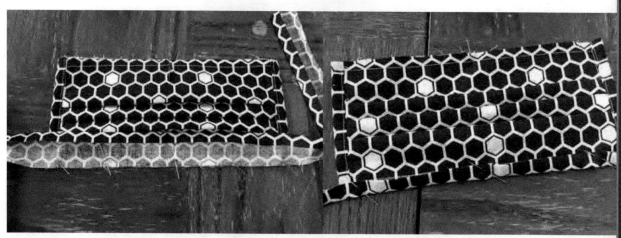

13. Unfold strap ends. Fold in 1/4", then re-fold pressed creases. Pin to secure

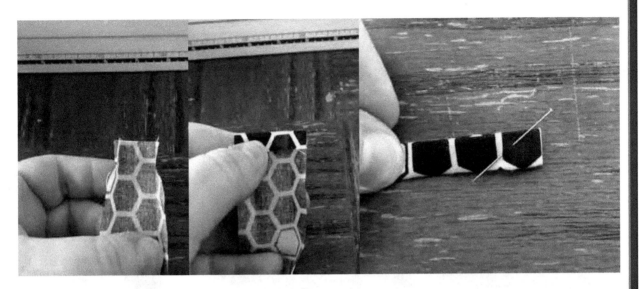

14. Top stitch along entire strap, including mask. To finish, stitch across strap ends to secure, and press pleats flat

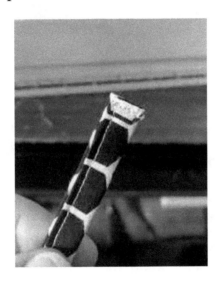

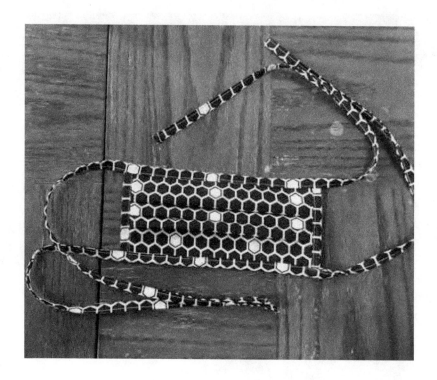
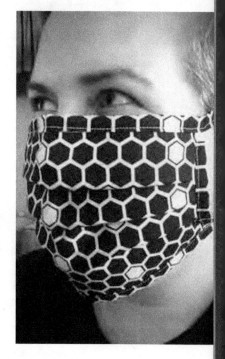

Three ways to upgrade the mask

We've shown you how to make a simple mask, based off of advice from the Pennsylvania Department of Health. But if you have a little more skill, here are three ways you can upgrade the mask:

Flip the mask inside-out instead of leaving the raw edges. Having the frayed edges inside could help keep the mask together and not degrade while being washed. It also looks nicer. To do this, first sew the ties to one layer, then layer the second layer on top of it. Then sew the two fabric layers together, leaving an inch or two of space instead of completing a full rectangle. Flip the mask inside-out through that rectangle, then sew around the outer edge again.

Fold horizontal pleats. This allows the mask to better fit the curvature of your face, similar to how surgical masks work. The New York Times has a guide to making a mask with pleats and that you flip inside-out.

Use a third layer. Experts recommend having two layers of material, but some designs use a third, disposable layer to help filter air even further. Those can include materials such as Swiffer disposable dusting pads, coffee filters, paper towels, or something similar, said Suzanne Willard, associate dean of global

DO IT YOURSELF HOMEMADE FACE MASK

health at Rutgers School of Nursing, who herself makes masks with disposable liners.

Some things to remember about your homemade mask

   Disinfect the mask between every use. The easiest way is to wash it with the rest of your laundry, in hot water and with soap or detergent, and then run it through the dryer. You may want to make more than one mask, depending how often you go outside.
   Take the mask off carefully. Wash your hands before taking the mask off and assume the virus is collected on the front of the mask. Don't touch the front directly, and instead take the mask off by the ties. Remember not to touch your face. Wash your hands after unmasking.

   Masks don't provide perfect protection. Wearing a mask does not give you more freedom to come in contact with others or otherwise engage in risky behaviors. Continue to stay home as much as you can and maintain physical distance from others when you do go outside.
   The mask should fit snugly around your nose and mouth. For an even better fit, you can sew a bendable piece of metal, such as a paperclip, to the top edge of the mask. That helps create a custom fit around the nose.

Do not touch the mask when in use, which risks transmitting the virus to your face.

Conclusion

Airborne diseases such as flu and COVID19 is spread from person-to-person in droplets of moisture, mucus and saliva from people with infections. Coughing, sneezing, and even normal breathing put these virus particles into the air. One sneeze can put out thousands of droplets.

People standing less than 6 feet away may become covered with these virus particles while they are still in the air. After the droplets fall, the virus particles can remain active for up to nine days.

Infection occurs when someone breathes in airborne droplets, or when they touch their mouth, nose or eyes with hands covered in virus particles that have fallen out of the air onto counters, hand rails, floors or other surfaces.

Wearing a face mask stops people from becoming infected in two ways:

1) By blocking most airborne droplets filled with virus from being inhaled

2) By stopping the wearer from touching their own mouths and noses.

Studies have shown that medical professional using surgical face masks correctly get 80% fewer infections than those who don't.

So why the mixed messages?

First, because the protection only comes when the masks are used properly. They must be put on clean, taken off carefully, and paired with rigorous hand washing, and the discipline not to touch the face.
Second, because gaps around the masks and between fibers, even in commercial surgical masks, are too large to block all viruses. Sneeze and cough droplets are usually between 7 and 100 microns. Surgical masks and some cloth masks will block 7 micron particles. The COVID19 virus particles are 0.06 to 0.14 microns.

So why should you make your own face masks?

1) In the event you become sick, having a supply of masks at home will give some level of protection to friends and family while you seek medical advice. It will certainly be better than no mask at all (see research notes).

2) By making your own, and hopefully for family and friends, you will be decreasing demand on limited supplies of industrially manufactured, disposables, which are desperately needed by hospitals and nursing homes.

3) These comfortable, curved shaped masks rest closer to the face, with fewer gaps, than rectangular surgical masks.

4) Our homemade designs are washable, making them environmentally friendly.

CPSIA information can be obtained
at www.ICGtesting.com
Printed in the USA
LVHW101240190121
676877LV00008B/367